26 Steps on the Road to Wellness

Laura M. Jacoby

Limits of Liability and Disclaimer of Warranty

The author and publisher shall not be liable for any misuse of this material. This book is strictly for informational and educational purposes.

Warning – Disclaimer

The purpose of this book is to inform, educate, and entertain. The author and/or publisher do not guarantee that anyone following these techniques, suggestions, tips, ideas, or strategies will become successful. The author and/or publisher shall have neither liability nor responsibility to anyone with respect to any loss or damage caused, or alleged to be caused, directly or indirectly, by the information contained in this book.

To my husband, my children, my grandchildren, and my special friends (you know who you are) for their love and support in helping me to visualize my wellness through the accomplishment of my dreams. I love you all so much!

A special thanks to my friend and editor, Lucy Spencer, without whom this would have not been possible.

LJ

Table of Contents

Preface

I never intended to write a book. This little book started out as my therapy in dealing with some personal family issues I was going through in the spring of 2013. I've always found that writing gives me closure and helps me to see beyond my problems. As April approached, I tried coming up with ways that I could help myself remember my own wellness steps, so I modeled the 26 Steps after the alphabet: A is for Action instead of apple, etc. For 26 days during the month of April, I wrote about these wellness steps in my blog. They gave me hope and something to look forward to instead of just dwelling on the problems I was facing at that time.

Each one of these steps is near and dear to my heart because it was through these 26 steps that I found a better way to live. While they're all intertwined with each other, each one can propel you into a new realm of living an abundantly happy life. It's interesting when we shake free from the shackles that hold us down, how much better we feel physically, emotionally, and spiritually. These steps helped me break free from my own shackles and moved me further on my journey to the person I was meant to be all along. No longer am I stuck in that same rut, on that same crazy-go-round, allowing what other people think of me hold me down.

From blog to book

I had the chance to go back over what I had written, and I could remember the day I wrote each post—what I was going through, and how far I had come. In rewriting Step 2, Building Bridges of Wellness, I realized that this is probably the most difficult one to accomplish but the most important to my wellness plan. I began asking myself questions like, "Do I say things to get a rise out of people?" "Do I push people's buttons?" "What is my part in the conflict that I have in my life?" These questions spurred me to understand the connection between my personal conflicts and my wellness.

When I understood this, I became more conscious of what motivates my actions.

This book is small in comparison to other self-help books. I'm not an expert in anything. I'm just an average middle-aged woman who has read and reread my favorite authors several times—Joyce Meyer, John C Maxwell, Zig Ziglar, Anthony Robbins, Stephen R. Covey, Dr. Caroline Leaf, and Sheila Walsh. Through these inspirational people, I've learned that we can change our lives if we are willing to do what's necessary.

I hope you will read through this entire book and think about how you can implement the steps, but I also hope these steps encourage you to find your own wellness steps. This book has no sequential chapters, so you're free to explore whichever step you feel you need most, whether it's Step 10, Journey to the Real You, or Step 16, Pete and Repeat. It doesn't matter where you are when you begin on your road to wellness. It's more important that you begin.

Introduction

Do you ever wonder why your life is not where you thought it would be? Most of us look at our lives in small compartments. We separate our family life from our health life, our work life from our social life, and we can't understand why we're so disconnected and unwell. When each component of a car's engine is working properly the car is easier to drive. The same is true for our life. When the components of our lives are working in harmony, life is not only easier but it's also filled with joyful abundance.

Life is as difficult as we make it out to be. Each of us is as unique as each snowflake that falls from the sky. We all have our set of likes, dislikes, tastes, and personalities that guide us through life as we want it to be. When you look through your own wellness steps, they are what make your life *your life*. Do you take a stroll at lunch time, or breathe deeply when in traffic? These are both wellness steps that many people use to help them get through their hectic days. But what if I told you that it's possible to memorize your Action Steps to Wellness as simply as you memorized the alphabet? Would you believe me?

Several of these steps include personal stories about my life, and how I overcame adversity to move past being a victim to being a survivor and a conqueror. (Just a word of warning: Step #11 follows no form at all.) At the end of each step is a quote that will help you remember the steps.

Some steps will address how you can apply that step to the seven realms of wellness—social, emotional, spiritual, environmental, occupational, intellectual, and physical—and answer these questions. How well do you connect with other people in your life?

- Your relationships with your family, your friends and your co-workers make up your social life. Can you make friends easily? Can you diffuse conflict when it arises within your social life?

- Adapting to life's constant changing circumstances means your emotional life is flourishing. Can you share your emotions in a constructive way?

- Harmony in life is the very core of the spiritual component. Are your values and actions harmonious to the purpose you have in life?

- Do you live an environmentally sound life? If you are constantly associating with unhealthy, negative people then you can't expect to have total wellness.

- How is your work life? Are you able to handle the stress at your workplace constructively?

- Do you engage in creative expression, or learn new things? Are you constantly growing and open to new ideas?

- Do you participate in some form of physical activity? How well do you sleep? How is your eating plan?

As you read this book, you will learn some basic, free, and low-cost ways to help your life's wholeness. You'll discover a new understanding about how to use the wellness choices that are available to you. You will also begin to see that your total wellness depends on the seven components of wellness (social, emotional, spiritual, environmental, occupational, intellectual, and physical) all working together.

When you put all of these 26 action steps to work in your own life, you'll begin to see that your wellness is in your own capable hands. While each step has its own merit, collectively they form a wellness plan that can propel you into a life you never thought was possible—a life filled with abounding health and magnificent wellness.

You are now cordially invited to check out Step 1, if you haven't already. Your wellness journey is about to begin, so hang on—you're in for one heck of a ride!

STEP 1: Action

When a movie director yells action, he wants the actors to fulfill the script and make a movie. Encarta Dictionary says that action is a movement, or doing something toward a goal. In order to accomplish our goals, we must act and do something.

How does this look in the real world?

- **Socially**: Do something to relate and connect with the people in your circle, your family, your coworkers, and your clients, if you run your own business. Write letters and make phone calls to the people in your life you want to thank, ask forgiveness, and just reconnect with.

- **Emotionally:** Act upon your own feelings. Show your feelings, but don't wear them on your sleeve. Give yourself permission to cry and feel sadness when needed. Ask yourself some important questions. "Am I filled with hope or stress?" "Do I share my feelings in an appropriate manner with my loved ones?" "Do I suck up my feelings and then gorge myself on chocolate, alcohol, or another addiction?" Once your feelings come out, you'll begin to experience a new sense of wellness.

- **Spiritually:** Pray, meditate, study the deeper meaning of life by filling your mind with our Creator's thoughts, and you'll be able to act in a different manner.

- **Environmentally:** Act responsible in your own environment. If you want to get off the crazy-go-round, then don't participate in the drama that surrounds it. If your desk is a mess, clean it up. If your home is a mess, clean it up. If your life is a mess, clean it up.

- **Occupationally:** If you're not doing your best at your job and just can't seem to get ahead, then do something to change it. If you're unemployed, start a small business or get career coaching. If you're at odds with your boss, sit down and try to iron out all the problems.

- **Intellectually:** Actively research new ideas and paths. Learning should be a lifelong joy. Make it a habit to learn something new each day and share that knowledge with the people in your life. If you have children, share what you learned at the dinner table.

- **Physically:** Do something today that will make your wellness tomorrow count. Exercise, pay attention to portion control, and try to eat only organic food. Stop the bad habits that are shortening your life.

"Do you want to know who you are? Don't ask. ACT! Action will delineate and define you."

Thomas Jefferson

STEP 2: Building Bridges of Wellness

Have you ever had an argument with yourself about what you should be doing but you're not? Many people go through this scenario and get frustrated with themselves instead of finding ways to get through the argument. When we're frustrated enough with a situation, we simply say, "Okay, enough! I'm not going to think about this anymore." Then we close the door and put a brick in front of it. Similarly, when we're having an argument with another person, the person may say, "We're not talking about this anymore." So we put another brick in the wall.

Instead of building bridges of wellness, we build walls of despair where we only have a handful of subjects that we can talk about. Eventually the walls get so tall that we can't see the other people in our lives.

Even arguments—the arguments in your own head—may stop you from building the bridges of wellness in your own life. You know, the arguments that start like this.

"You're too old to do this!"

"Remember what happened last time you tried something like this?"

"You're in too much pain."

"Just go back to bed."

These are like the drain stoppers in the sink. Statements like these drain you of any movement forward, and they stop you from becoming the person you can be.

There's always a place to build a bridge in your own life. An example of this comes from my marriage. I remember when my husband and I were first married and we were having a disagreement. My husband just stopped talking; he looked at me and told me he loved me. It melted my heart. His loving words built a bridge between us.

How do we build bridges of wellness on the job? If you hate your job, find something you love about it. Focus on that one thing you love about your career, and soon your bridge will be done and you may even find that you love your job. Every time you choose to build bridges of wellness over building walls of despair, your health grows stronger and your life grows more peaceful.

"I like to see myself as a bridge builder that is me building bridges between people, between races, between cultures, between politics, trying to find common ground."

T. D. Jakes

STEP 3: Commit to Creating Your Life

Has your life ever been on autopilot, where you just go through the motions each day but fail to actually connect to your day? Each day when you open your eyes, you get a "do-over"—another chance to create the kind of life you want. But so many of us are stuck on autopilot, with blinders on, only looking at the fringes of what our lives could be instead of choosing to commit to creating our lives! How committed are you to creating your life?

You know the drill...the alarm goes off, you shuffle to the coffee maker, push a button, you brush your teeth, you get dressed, you fix your hair, you grab your coffee, and you head out the door. That's called autopilot. You can do these things with your eyes closed. If you have kids to care for, then you have one eye open but you're still on autopilot. You see, when you put your life on autopilot, you've willingly given up control and whatever happens in your life will control your life instead of you having a say in creating the life you want.

When you commit to creating your life, you don't need an alarm to wake you up; you get up naturally. You don't need coffee to get you going in the morning; you're energized because you had a restful night. There's no need to go back to bed when the kids go off to school, because you can't wait to get started on all the exciting things you have planned. If you keep dreaming of what your life could be, if only...then you're not committed to creating the life you want to have.

Stop dreaming of "if only" and start committing to creating your life the way you want it. Yes, it's going to be difficult at times. No one said it would be easy! Without your never-ending commitment, your life will be filled with "what if."

"What if I had stuck with that exercise and diet plan?"

"What if I didn't give up?"

"What if I worked on that relationship a little more?"

Each day you wake up with a clean slate; do something different. If you always have coffee for breakfast, have a protein shake instead. If you go back to bed after the kids leave for school, stay up and work out, go for a walk, or talk to someone. If weight loss is something you're seeking, stop eating one processed meal a day and substitute it with an organic salad. If you think you made a mistake somewhere along your life, go back and apologize and start over. If owning a business is on your mind, do some research and find where your interests lie and go for it.

If you're still breathing, you have another chance to make it right.

"Trust yourself. Create the kind of self that you will be happy to live with all your life. Make the most of yourself by fanning the tiny, inner sparks of possibility into flames of achievement."

Golda Meir

STEP 4: Decide What You Want and Go After It

How many times have you started a wellness plan, weight loss program, or workout routine and then grew bored and stopped cold? Many times we've gone through this cycle where we make a decision to do something, do it for a month, and when it gets difficult, we stop. Instead of stopping next time, push through the obstacles that come along to derail your decision about what you want.

Deciding looks like this:

- **Social:** Do you want better relationships with your family? Be open to different ways of bringing the family together. Facilitate the healing process by being accessible and approachable to all your family members. Seek professional help if the rifts are too big to handle on your own.

- **Emotional:** Know your reasons for wanting what you want, because they will help you to deal with certain life stresses that will still be present. Share your feelings and anxieties when they arise instead of hiding them inside, where they do more damage.

- **Spiritual:** Can't figure out what you want? Pray about it. Meditate about it. The answers will come and when they do, you'll know exactly what needs to get done in order to experience the joy of deciding!

- **Occupational:** If you're not getting what you want from your career or job, there are always ways to fix it. But if you're not really sure what you want, you'll never get it. Figure out what you want: more money, more free time, more time to be creative. If your performance is high, chances are you may only have to *ask* for what you want. If not, do whatever is ethically necessary to reach your goal.

- **Intellectual:** When you open yourself up to different opportunities, you'll be amazed at how much this helps you decide what you really want. This could include attending free seminars on subjects that interest you. Health clubs and health food stores frequently give free health seminars. Book stores often invite an author to speak about his or her book. Local libraries offer book readings. Look around your community to see what you may be missing.

- **Physical:** Deciding to lose weight and getting healthy are two of the top decisions a person makes in life, along with getting married, changing careers, going to school, moving to a new city, starting a business, and having children.

"Being the richest man in the cemetery doesn't matter to me. Going to bed at night saying we've done something wonderful, that's what matters to me."

Steve Jobs

STEP 5: Educate Yourself

When a child enters kindergarten, he or she is not expected to know everything, or the teachers would not have a job. With each new grade level, a child learns more and more, and by the time the child graduates from high school, he or she knows more than how to read and write. Our education doesn't stop when we graduate, as many people think. To expand our horizons and open the doors of opportunity, we need to continually educate ourselves.

When we live our lives in stagnancy, we close off the world around us without even knowing it. Through educating ourselves, we break free from the closed-off box we built for ourselves and we experience life to a fuller degree. No more are we just shining our lights in our own little box and only blinding ourselves.

Ways to educate yourself:

- **Workshops:** If you want to learn how to build something, cook, start a new craft, repair something, or take better care of yourself, check out your favorite home improvement stores, craft stores, kitchen gadget stores, or health food stores. They usually post new workshops online and in their stores.

- **YouTube:** A wealth of information can be learned here from people who are actually doing it, including what works and what doesn't.

- **Mentors:** This is one of the best ways to learn new skills, especially when you're in business. Mentors are assets to success because they not only want you to succeed, but they will motivate you to be a better you.

- **Seminars and Webinars:** A wealth of information can be learned from these sources as well. They are given by experts in their field: doctors, naturopaths, chiropractors, network marketers, authors—the list goes on and on.

- **Friends:** How many times have you run to your friends and said, "You're really good at this or that, can you teach me how to do it?" How many times have your friends wanted to share what they are learning with you? Don't shut the door on them. You may just have found another way to educate yourself.

"Education is the most powerful weapon which you can use to change the world."

Nelson Mandela

STEP 6: Find What Works

Media is constantly telling us that the newest diet craze is the best one out there and everyone should be on it. You need to remember that the media is all about ratings and selling what's hot at the moment. As a consumer, you need to find what works best for your own body and your own lifestyle, and just do it.

The following is an example that will help you understand why it's so important to find what works for your own life.

Heart disease runs in my family. My doctor told me that eating a fat-free vegan diet would reduce my risk of having heart disease. I lived on a vegan diet for several years, but I always felt like I was missing something: good healthy fat. So I did some research, and I found out why I was constantly having brain fog and memory loss issues. My brain needed fat.

An adult human brain is made up of 60% fat.[1] So if we're not eating good fats, then our brains are starving because they need the fat to assimilate fat-soluble vitamins and minerals. When I decided to add organic chicken and wild-caught fish, I began thinking better and my memory was not the problem it once was. My skin also looked and felt better after adding high-quality fats such as organic, cold-pressed coconut oil, olive oil, walnut oil, and flax oil. I still eat a vegan diet four days a week, but I make a conscious effort to choose foods that help me and my body.

Take the time to find what works for your own wellness. Do some research. Ask questions. Just as your fingerprints are unique to you, your personal wellness is unique. Find what works for you and do it.

This is not just about your health; it's about your life. The point is to be the best person you can be and don't let people or the media walk all over you. When you find your niche in life, your whole life will open up with possibilities! You'll begin to see things differently, and you'll find that you like yourself a whole lot more when you are *you* and not trying to fit into a mold that someone else has created for you.

"Look, all you can do when you find your niche is go with it."

Vincent D. Onofrio

STEP 7: Give Yourself a Chance

The moment you get sick with a cold is the moment when you start drowning all your symptoms in hopes that they will all just disappear in time for you to go to work, school, or a recreational activity. It's interesting to note that people will begin taking better care of themselves only after they have been given a bad report from the doctor. They want their risks of diseases lowered instantly, but that's not how wellness works. You need to give yourself a chance to grow in wellness throughout your life, not just for a day, a week, a month, or even a year.

Each time you reach for those nighttime and daytime cold medicines, you are also ingesting harmful chemicals, such as artificial coloring and flavoring and alcohol. These chemicals stop the healing process. Coughing and sneezing are cold symptoms that allow our bodies to loosen and expel the mucus that the germs are producing. Taking a medicine that stops the healing process only pushes the infection deeper into our bodies. The same is true for an alcoholic who drowns his or her sorrows with alcohol instead of dealing with the emotions they are trying to mask.

Alternative remedies that give your body a chance to heal while strengthening your immune system:

- **ASEA**: This product makes everything else in this arsenal of cold remedies work better. Taken twice a day, it will help the body to do what it's supposed to when fighting off illnesses.[2]

- **Elderberry**: Drink as a tea or as an elixir. It is good for colds and flu.[3]

- **Fenugreek:** Drink as a tea. It loosens mucus.[4]

- **Feverfew**: Taken in tincture form, it's great for headaches of any kind—even migraines.[5]

- **Garlic**: Eat whole and raw. Its properties are potent enough to get rid of many germs, and even some people you don't want around you.[6]

- **Lemon Juice**: The fresh juice of one lemon added to a cup of boiling water sweetened with honey will help break up the mucus. This mixture will also help the body to remain more alkaline, which in turn helps you stay healthy because illness loves an acid environment.[7]

- **Oil of Oregano**: Take in drops. Four drops under the tongue three times a day has the power to knock out any infection. It's a strong, natural antibiotic.[8]

Each step in of your wellness journey is filled with choices of how you treat yourself and other people. It's a known fact that what you give to others will come back to you. You can't love your neighbor unless you love yourself.

"One's philosophy is not best expressed in words; it is expressed in the choices one makes...and the choices we make are ultimately our responsibility."

Eleanor Roosevelt

STEP 8: Hear Me Now

Each day when you wake up, your body is telling you that it has had enough sleep and is ready to start the day. As a matter of fact, your body is constantly trying to tell you something, only you don't hear it, or you choose to ignore what you hear. Your health and wellness depends on how well you listen to what your body is telling you.

The biggest problem is not in the listening so much as it is in what you choose to hear. Remember watching the Verizon commercial where the guy is going into remote places and asking, "Can you HEAR me now?" Think about how your body is screaming this to you every chance it can, while you turn a deaf ear and continue on your not-so-merry way.

The difference between hearing and listening to your body is as clear as night and day. My husband's way of dealing with pain is a great example of this. He was in a bicycle accident several years ago. When I got to the emergency room where he was taken, I heard him having harsh words with the nurse because he didn't want any pain meds. The nurse kept insisting and my husband held his ground. His final statement on the matter has been a continual reason why he will never take pain meds: "I need to know what my body is doing, and pain meds cover up what's going on inside me!"

This brings up another point of hearing what your body is saying. For two years now my husband and I have been trying to get rid of all the wheat from our diet, because it's so genetically modified and because my husband has gluten *intolerance*. So I did some research and found that spelt flour is not as modified and people who are gluten-intolerant can sometimes do fine on it.[9] So I used spelt flour in everything and played around with alternative flours (tapioca, brown rice, and garbanzo bean). About a month ago, I stopped using the spelt altogether and just used the tapioca, brown rice, and garbanzo bean.

Something wonderful has happened with my husband's health issues. They've gone away. My husband heard what his body was saying every time he would eat something that had gluten in it. He was able to listen to what he heard his body telling him. Yesterday while eating my cornbread made with garbanzo bean flour, he said that he has no problem eating this way, and he feels so much better.

If you smoke and you're constantly sick with respiratory problems (colds, flu, sinus infections, allergies, or chronic bronchitis), your lungs are screaming at you[10], "Can you HEAR me now?" Don't wait until you have lung cancer, emphysema, or COPD to listen to it. HEAR what your body is saying NOW.

If you're having scaly or blotchy skin issues, your body is trying to tell you that you have a food allergy or sensitivity.[11] There are two ways to determine if you have food allergies or sensitivities: you could either go into your doctor and have the blood and scratch test or you can do the elimination diet.[12] The offending foods that trigger these skin issues and should be eliminated are dairy, citrus fruits, tomatoes, soy, shellfish, eggs, wheat, and gluten.[13] HEAR what your body is saying instead of trying to cover up the problem with lotions and makeup.

Instead of running to the medicine cabinet to get rid of every discomfort—heartburn, headaches, skin rashes, etc.— learn to listen to what your body is trying to tell you. Each of these discomforts is a warning sign that something is amiss in your body. If you're constantly covering up the discomforts of life, you stop yourself from hearing what your body is saying. It's like ignoring a blaring smoke alarm. You wouldn't ignore the smoke alarm at work, school, or in your own home; you would do whatever is necessary to find out where the smoke was coming from. Stop ignoring the alarms your body is blaring at you.

"My back talks to me in the only way it can, using symbols – symptoms – making me aware of an embedded story."

Dr. Dawn Garisch

STEP 9: Imagine

Do you ever sit back and just think of what could be? As a child, you probably imagined all the time, but when you started getting in trouble for daydreaming, you probably stopped imagining how life could be and became a little robot like the rest of the children, going about your day on autopilot. It's time to start imagining again.

Imagine how your life could be with the application of one of these steps. In pursuing a new career, job seekers are constantly asked that ill-fated question: "Where do you see yourself in five years?" If you can't see what your life would be like in five years, it's because you haven't imagined what it could be like.

Baby steps to the rescue.

- **Imagine** what tomorrow would be like if you changed just one thought or one action. If you're constantly putting yourself down, image how you would feel tomorrow if you complimented yourself on your good habits. ("Tomorrow when I pass by a mirror I will say, 'Hello Gorgeous!' I can see myself smiling.") If driving in traffic causes you stress, imagine how tomorrow would be different if you listened to a good book or soothing music while you drove. Do this for a month, and you'll see life a whole lot differently.

- **Imagine** how a certain color would change your attitude. Do you wear black most of the time? Imagine how your attitude might change if you bring more color into your home, your wardrobe, and your life. Now imagine bringing in some pretty flowers for your table and see how it affects your attitude. (For two weeks, I wore clothes with colors other than black and it lightened my mood and my attitude!)

- **Imagine** you are surrounded by positive, influential people within your chosen career or interest. You're having a conversation with them; imagine what you would be saying and what you would be learning.

- **Imagine** what your version of happiness looks like and think about that all the time. When you think happy thoughts, you become happy, no matter what's going on in your life.

- **Keep on imagining** and seeing yourself in two weeks, a month, and even a year. What are you doing? What are you wearing? Who's with you? How will your life be better?

When you imagine, you open up your world to the possibilities in life. Can you see the possibilities in your life? If not, then you're not imagining enough!

"Imagination is everything. It is the preview of life's coming attractions."

Albert Einstein

STEP 10: Journey into the Real You

When was the last time you ventured out of your comfort zone? You can't find a fulfilling life in the easy chair of life. Journeying into the real you goes deeper than just finding out what you like and don't like about yourself and your life. It's all about how truthful you are to the people you love and respect.

Journeying into your real self takes time, patience, research, and love. Taking the time to find out what character traits you love in yourself and other people depends on whether you are able to overlook faults, because it is in overlooking other people's faults where you begin to see what you overlook in yourself.

There is a long-standing principle that when you act like yourself, you are happier. This is true because you aren't trying to be someone else, but you're embracing the real you. When two people get married and one of them is trying to change the other person into someone they aren't, then the marriage is doomed from the beginning. Changing yourself is a whole lot easier than trying to change other people.

You'll need to take the journey of experiences that you've never had before. As a child, your parent probably had you try different foods by telling you, "If you try it, you might like it." Did your parent know you'd like it? Probably not, but that was their way of getting you to try a new taste palate. Perhaps you've always disliked a certain food but had to eat it because it was on your plate, and throughout your life you just tolerated it. It's time to stop doing that. You don't have to eat food you don't like or participate in activities that aren't you just because it's something you've always done.

It takes research to find the real you. Sometimes you put your hopes and dreams on the back burner because life took over; you got married, had kids, and lost yourself in the process. If your children are grown, it's time to bring the real you out, the one your spouse fell in love with.

If you are truthful to the real you, you'll be truthful to the people around you. You'll be able to handle the stresses of life better when you're *you*. If you're looking for happiness and it seems to elude you, try journeying into the real you. Follow Shakespeare's advice: "To thine own self be true."

How?

- Stop lying to yourself and to everyone else. What you put out to the world comes back to you.

- Stop exaggerating the stories of your life. Tell your story, but don't make it a tall tale.

- Stop overreacting to situations in life. Simply let go of the reins and realize that you'll never be able to control anyone but yourself.

"Always be a first-rate version of yourself and not a second-rate version of someone else."

Judy Garland

STEP 11: Keep It Going

Since you want to make a consistent effort to be the best version of you possible you need to keep doing certain things that will motivate you to be positive when times get tough.

Keep breathing. Keep smiling. Keep moving. Keep shining. Keep dreaming. Keep imagining. Keep planning. Keep laughing. Keep deciding where you want to go. Keep giving yourself a chance. Keep paying it forward. Keep singing. Keep dancing. Keep running. Keep reading. Keep asking. Keep doing. Keep sharing. Keep saving. Keep encouraging. Keep inspiring. Keep writing. Keep helping. Keep praying. Keep serving. Keep listening. Keep searching. Keep your eyes open. Keep finding. Keep learning. Keep playing. Keep loving. Keep speaking. Keep hearing. Keep watching. Keep bringing. Keep painting. Keep creating. Keep keeping it real. Keep telling the truth. Keep natural. Keep organic.

Keep living in the present. Keep changing. Keep growing. Keep putting one foot in front of the other. Keep improving. Keep showing up. Keep forgiving. Keep calling. Keep compassion in your life. Keep empathy a part of your life. Keep thinking. Keep camping. Keep hiking. Keep climbing. Keep walking. Keep swimming. Keep hugging. Keep your lamp burning. Keep spinning. Keep digging. Keep eating healthy food. Keep taking your supplements. Keep cooking. Keep sowing. Keep harvesting. Keep pruning. Keep mentoring. Keep building bridges. Keep tearing down walls. Keep recommitting. Keep appreciating. Keep standing. Keep feeling. Keep making peace. Keep staying positive. Keep praising. Keep journaling. Keep journeying into reality. Keep promising. Keep coaching. Keep making love. Keep kissing.

Keep it going!

"If you're going through hell, keep going."

Winston Churchill

STEP 12: Leave the Past Behind

Some people go through hell and back in their life and live to talk about it, while others are consumed by the hurt, the pain, and the anger that is associated with their childhood or other life experiences. These people who have been able to leave the past behind are more resilient than those who carry their past with them.

We all have a past. My past was dotted with tragedy. My best friend died of leukemia when I was six. I never understood that because no one ever took the time to explain it to me.

Then there was the constant torment of my other brother; he would hold my head under water, and make me feel like I was worthless and make me think I was adopted all the time.

My mom used to yell at me instead of just talking to me like a normal person (I'm not sure why she yelled).

Then there were the crazy things I did as a teenager that put me in dangerous situations. One of them involved a gun pointed up against my temple when I walked into a store that was in the process of being robbed. You know, the things you never told your parents.

Then at the age of 19, I was abused by a family member, who told me that if I told anyone he would just say I was lying and the family would believe him over me anyway.

Being pregnant with twins (a boy and a girl) and having a miscarriage when I was five and a half months pregnant, I felt like it was my fault that I miscarried my daughter.

My father died when I was 25 and, while I was crying over it, I was told, "Buck up. You have nothing to cry over."

I'm sure there are some of you reading this who know what it's like to be abused and be too fearful to tell anyone. As I look back over what's happened in my life, I should have said something. I should have gone to the police and let the blame fall where it was supposed to. But I let myself become the victim instead of becoming the strong woman of faith I could have been.

Many times, this one incident has led me to be afraid of the things I shouldn't be afraid of in life. I dared not go places by myself. I'm sometimes still nervous in a roomful of people (I tend to walk the perimeter of the room, knowing where all the exits are). I don't feel comfortable meeting men for the first time without my husband. The list is endless.

I am also a firm believer that our nerves hold memories of what we've gone through in life, like a memory chip storing data. When more life stress or horrendous news like the Boston Marathon Bombings or the tornadoes in Oklahoma gets piled on top of what we already have, those nerve memories are stirred up and our body responds by giving us unexplained pain, nausea, fear, insomnia, digestive issues, anxiety, blood pressure issues, and everything in between.

I've made peace with my past, and you can too. I forgave all the people in my life that have caused me extreme pain, but that doesn't mean I want to have a relationship with them. In order to have some semblance of sanity, you need to leave the past behind, leave the toxic people in the past, and leave the anger about "Why did this happen?" in the past.

Growing, maturing, and changing involve coming to grips with your past and just plain saying, "Enough is enough!" The past only holds you there as long as you let it. Leave your past behind. Your present and your future will not only thank you, but they will open up the best possibilities that life has to offer.

"People who live in the past generally are afraid to compete in the present. I've got my faults, but living in the past is not one of them. There's no future in it."

Sparky Anderson

STEP 13: Make a Difference

How often have you been told that, in order to change your own life and your own outlook on life, you need to make a difference in someone else's life?

You need to make a difference in your own life first. It's easy to make a difference in other people's lives, but oh-so-difficult to make that same difference in your own life. When you make a difference in your own life, your life becomes what you want it to be, and you are better able to make a difference in the lives of the people around you.

To make a difference in your own life, you need to change your mindset about what makes you happy, how you need to be really sick and tired of how your life is, how you need to be totally uncomfortable about sitting on the edge of your life instead of participating in it.

Ways you can make a difference in your own life:

- Make a date with yourself every day to read or listen to an inspirational message. Read your Bible, and listen to different ministries (one of my favorites is http://livingontheedge.org).

- Try reading while exercising on a stationary bike or listening while going for a walk.

- Make it a point to do something encouraging in your own life. Put up inspirational quotations around your home or office. Tape some of them to your bathroom mirror or your refrigerator. You can even frame some of them to hang in prominent places so you can see them when you least expect to.

- Surround yourself with people who are encouraging, supportive, loving, and kind. Not all of the people in your life are here to encourage you; some are here to teach you how *not* to behave. There will always be people in your lives who are ready to whip you around with their tongues, but you don't have to listen to them or be around them. You'll make a difference in your own life if you distance yourself from these kinds of people.

- What we think about, we bring about. So, to make a difference in your own life, change how you think. Stop using curse words. Think about the good things in life, even though you may be going through difficult times. Stop dwelling on the negative. In looking for the good, the silver lining, you open yourself up to the best possibilities that life can offer.

- Think about what and how you eat. If being positive and inspiring is one of your goals, then you have to eat better food. Clean, organic food is the only way to supply your brain and body with the nutrients it needs to accomplish your daily challenges. Plus, it helps you think better, which in turn helps you make better choices.

"Believe in yourself! Have faith in your abilities! Without a humble buy reasonable confidence in your own powers you cannot be successful or happy."

Norman Vincent Peale

STEP 14: Nourish Your Own Life

Each part of your life needs nourishment. A brain cannot function properly without the necessary nutrients to help it perform on a daily basis. This is also true for every other body organ. Proper nourishment in your life will not only help you live a better life, but it will also propel you forward in your search for what you want and need in your life.

If you're filling your life with negative forces and vibrations, then your life will be filled with everything you don't want. But if you turn the knob and change what you think about, you'll be able to nourish your life, and your life will be filled with what you want. Happiness is good for your heart and great for your health.

Some simple ways to nourish your life

- Go on a negativity fast. For seven days, don't allow anything negative to come into your life or out of your mouth. Try to get away from the negative people in your life. It's just for seven days. Then write about your experiences and how your life is different after the seven days compared to the time before you started.

- During those seven days, read books written by John C. Maxwell, Zig Ziglar, Joyce Meyer, Dale Carnegie, Tony Robbins, Brian Tracy, etc. Fill your minds with uplifting movies—*Fireproof*, *Facing the Giants*, and *Courageous* are just a few of them.

- Stop using curse words. What comes out of your mouth has a direct relationship to what's in your heart.

- Reconnect with nature. Go on a hike or a walk in a park. Listen to the birds singing and the children playing. Walk barefoot in the grass or the sand. Let your whole being connect with the earth. It's calming, soothing, and rejuvenating all at the same time.

- Clean out your living space. A nourished life thrives in an organized home. Your home is a reflection of what's inside you. Get rid of things that are just taking up space that you have no attachments to. You'll be amazed at how freeing it is when you do this.

- Clean out your refrigerator and your pantry. Get rid of all the processed food and begin to eat a clean diet. Know what goes into your food. Processed food is another form of negativity because it has a negative effect on your body.

These are clearly not the easiest tasks you'll ever face, but when you do, they will help you to nourish every part of your life.

"Your health runs on happiness!"

Laura Jacoby

STEP 15: Open Your Eyes

Everyone seems to be searching for that miracle cure that will let them continue with their unhealthy lifestyle, yet make them invincible when it comes to diseases. The miracle cure for most diseases is you. You are the miracle prevention, you are the miracle cause, and you are the miracle cure. Just open your eyes and you'll see that what you've been thinking, doing, and eating are all contributors to either great health or devastatingly bad health.

It's really simple. If you think bad thoughts all the time and walk around with a negative attitude, your body will follow suit and become energetically blocked. Negative thoughts not only kill your attitudes, but they change your genes and your cells so you are more susceptible to contracting devastating diseases and illnesses. But the opposite—positive thoughts—can actually help people overcome those diseases. If you change your negative thoughts to positive ones, then the diseases won't get a foothold in your body.

Here's something to think about: if you carry a lot of anger around with you on a daily basis and you notice that you're in more pain than usual, try letting go of the anger and see if the pain also goes away. It may take a bit of time, but this one change could affect the rest of your life.

Whatever you think about—positive or negative—you end up doing. So if you are thinking negatively or swearing at those whom you say you love, you are actively taking those negative thoughts and giving them permission to run your lives by your actions.

Think about it. Negative thoughts left unchecked will ruin your entire day. Imagine the scenario: on your way to work someone cuts you off in traffic, instead of letting it go you say a couple of curse words. Then your favorite barista at the coffee house gets your coffee order wrong, and you speak to her very harshly. "I've ordered the same drink every morning for the last two years. How can you get my order wrong?" Then walking into your office, you spill your coffee all over your new suit. That negative thought you had when someone cut you off on your way to work was the catalyst that snowballed into your negative day. Days like that will continue to spiral out of control, until you reel in your negative thoughts.

"I'm not worth it!"

"I'm no good!"

"No one loves me!"

"Get out of my life!"

So when you think those things, you're setting the stage for that very thing to happen. Telling yourself you're not worth it, you're no good, or no one loves you will put you into situations where those words come true.

An example from my own life helps explain this even further. I used to tell myself all sorts of lies like "I'm no good!" and "I can't do anything right!" I acted on them, too, by trying to satiate my feelings with food, procrastination, sleep, and, yes, anger at myself. Then one day, with the help of a friend, I began to realize what I was doing in my life. So I just stopped the lies. I asked God to help me change my thoughts to only think of the positive, and it happened—not instantly, but gradually. It's freeing to look at only the positive side of situations. It's helped my life, my marriage, my family, and my health.

If you can't stand to be around phony people, then why would you stuff your mouths and your lives with phony food that robs your bodies of nutrients instead of giving you what you need and want most? We cannot eat fake, GMO food and expect to be healthy. Is it too difficult to understand that you hold the key to your own health in the choices you make about food? Sometimes people like living under a rock because then they won't be responsible for what they know. I've had many people tell me they don't want to know what's lurking in their food—they are happy in their oblivion. These are the same people that are always asking for suggestions on how they can help their families be healthier.

Then there is the other side of the coin, where you think you have a disease, and you do so much research that you start manifesting symptoms of the disease. You even print out documentation to give to the many doctors you visit to help them do their jobs in making the diagnosis that you've convinced yourself you have.

This is not to say that using the Internet to research an illness you already have or are being tested for is not a good idea, because it is. The problem is in too much information also known as information overload. This information overload comes from listening to all the media doctors, nutritionists, dieticians, and health blog writers and trying to decipher what's real information and what is just plain garbage or personal choice. Who can you believe, when one day these media doctors are debunking the benefits of coffee and the next day they're touting coffee's benefits to make their sponsors happy?

There is only one way to gain the knowledge that *you* need, and that's doing research on your own. For instance, doctors and health specialists are now saying that processed food should be eliminated from diets because it is slowly killing people.[14] You can Google this and get all different kinds of website articles and blog posts, but you can also click the "MORE" tab and research different books that take aim at this target.

Some websites are more reliable than others. The National Institutes of Health is a reliable website, but they offer only what is deemed conventional methods and will only direct queries to government-sponsored health websites. Wikipedia is never considered a reliable source by most colleges and researchers because the information is allowed to be published without necessarily being verified.

When talking about subjects such as how processed foods are hurting the human race, I recommend books by top doctors like Dr. Russell L. Blaylock, who wrote *Excitotoxins: The Taste That Kills*. If you want to know how to reverse three of the major illnesses plaguing people today, I suggest that you check the writings and websites of Dr. Joel Fuhrman and Dr. Mark Hyman. To learn more about genetically modified foods, I would go to the people who have spent their entire lives doing the research, such as Jeffrey Smith of the Institute for Responsible Technology.

"Open your eyes so you can be the miracle prevention and the miracle cure instead of the miracle cause."

Laura Jacoby

STEP 16: Pete and Repeat

How many times have you heard this favorite children's joke: "Pete and Repeat are in a boat, Pete fell out, who was left?" And you go around in circles with the child, telling the joke. But there's a principle in that little joke, and it goes like this. If you keep repeating the same words, actions, and habits, you'll get the same results and you'll get stuck in a loop. Once you change the answer, the whole joke changes. Once you change a habit, your whole life changes.

Albert Einstein was a wise man. He said, "Insanity: doing the same thing over and over again and expecting different results." But what if you took the tool of repetition and used it to your advantage? You could change your life with little effort, and you'll make a lasting influence on your future generations.

What you repeat in your head is your driving force for your days. If you wake up in the morning and have no driving force, or you don't even make it out of bed, then it's beyond time to repeat some different words.

If all that your mind hears is "I'm FAT!" "I'm UGLY!", then your body will follow suit. It's very difficult to smile when you tell yourself you're ugly or fat. Your body will respond by making what you say come true. If you keep walking around with "I'm FAT!" playing in your head, then you will choose foods that will make you fat, and your body will become fat—or fatter. But you can change your mind just by changing your words.

Some daily phrases to help you move past the insanity:

- 2 Day is GR8!

- I'm active and I love it!

- I lead a healthy, pain-free life!

- I am beautiful on the inside and on the outside!

- My muscles are here to stay!

- Fat just keeps falling off me!

- I am loveable!

- I am beautiful!

- I am energized!

"You affect your subconscious mind by verbal repetition."

W. Clement Stone

STEP 17: Quiet Your Mind

Sometimes the only way to make sense of your world and your wellness is to quiet your mind. The instant world is always on. Social media is becoming the big brother of storybooks. Your entire life is posted for the world to read with your friends reporting every movement you make. It's become the place where you seek approval with "likes, comments, and shares."

To lead a quiet life, you need to unchain yourself from the ties that bind you to the very things that are sucking the life right out of you and your family. Your quiet life hangs in the balance when your life can be turned upside down by something as simple as a tweet that someone posted about you.

Quieting the mind has more to do with what you allow in your mind than with just turning off technology. Once you turn off technology, what do you do? Read a book, take a nap, sing your own songs, dance around your house, or have a picnic in the living room. Talk to your family, talk to your pet, and cuddle up by the fire. Enjoy the stillness without the sound vibrations from your electronics.

Quiet your mind by taking public transportation to work instead of driving yourself. Put your cell phone in your purse or your pocket and make a commitment to leave it there. Look out the window; let your mind wander and daydream. Talk to the person next to you. Read a book of poetry. Listen to the sounds of the city instead of the sounds of the texts and e-mails.

Quiet your mind while at work. Get up and move away from your desk at least twice every two hours. During your lunch break, take a therapeutic walk outside with no electronics. Just breathe in the fresh air.

Quiet your mind while walking outside with no headphones in your ears. Just listen to the wind. Say hello to people you pass. Listen to the leaves as they sway in the breeze.

Quiet your mind by breathing in all of the calmness and breathing out all of the negative emotions you've encountered. I was a sickly child and was always being poked with needles. One nurse showed me how to overcome the pain of the needles. While the needle was entering my arm, I inhaled very slowly and rhythmically. As the needle was coming out, I exhaled very slowly. It worked when I was 17 and it still works today.

"The best cure for the body is a quiet mind."

Napoleon Bonaparte

STEP 18: Raise Your Expectations

The world says that if you want to be happy, you'll have to lower your standards and your expectations of other people and yourself. That is not the path to wellness.

If you've spent time lowering your expectations and accepting only the minimal from the people around you, and you're still not happy, then it's time to turn it all around. If you raise your expectations, people will rise to meet them, and you'll do the same thing.

It's funny how the world tells you that in order to be happy, you need to lower your expectations of other people and of yourself. But when you lower your expectations, you're telling other people that you don't really matter and you give them license to treat you any way they want to. Plus, when you lower the expectations in your own life, you die a little to yourself.

If you don't matter to you, you won't matter to other people.

How do you raise your expectations?

- Set goals for yourself—achievable goals—with tasks attached to each goal. If you haven't set goals in a while, think about what you have accomplished without any goals. Not much, huh? Now think about what you want to accomplish. These goals will help you see what you need to do to reach the next level.

- Get out of your comfort zone, even if it means you have to burn your easy chair or give it to charity. You know what makes you uncomfortable. Are you uncomfortable speaking in front of large groups of people? Are you uncomfortable calling people and inviting them to look at your service? Are you uncomfortable being a peacemaker? Are you uncomfortable doing things on your own? When you get out of your comfort zone, you raise the bar on your own life, you expand your horizons, and you raise your expectations.

- Challenge yourself to do something different. Greatness is learned by people who challenge themselves to do and be different than the crowd. If the crowd is all running in the same direction, turn around and go the other way. Yes, it might feel like you're going upstream, and the people around you might even try to push you backward. But stand firm and move forward. The challenges can be as simple as challenging yourself to smile at least 10 times a day, if you're not prone to smiling. Every time you accomplish the little challenges, you move toward raising your expectations of what you can accomplish in your life.

"If you paint in your mind a picture of bright and happy expectations, you put yourself into a condition conducive to your goal."

Norman Vincent Peale

STEP 19: Serve It Up

Business success is totally dependent on how well clients and customers are served. If you do a good job, you may make a sale, but you may also make a friend.

You serve people all day long without even knowing it. Whether you think about it or not, you pay for good service more than anything else. Think about the wait staff who bend over backwards to make your dining experience the best and accommodate your dietary restrictions.

Serving people helps you take a break from your own life to focus on others.

Serving people is not a platform to look for reward or fame; it shouldn't be like the celebrities who are always serving organizations to get free publicity. Serving should come from your heart and focus on the person you are serving, not on how you look. It should be a blessing in your life to know that what you do makes an impact on the lives of the people you serve, and that reward should be enough for you.

When you serve, it should be a direct extension of who you are. Take yourself out of the picture when you're serving, and it will help you focus on other people's issues. It will also help you to see other people's strengths and ways to use those strengths in your own life.

Ways you can serve the people in your community, your church, and your family:

- **Volunteer** at a local Boys & Girls Club. Be a mentor to children who need a positive role model in their lives.

- **Help** out at the local food bank or food pantry. Anyone can write a check or donate food, but it takes a special person to physically help people in need.

- **Volunteer** at a senior center to play cards, do crafts, or just plain talk to the senior citizens who have given much and have much more to give.

- **Make** a plan to pray for each of your friends near and far. Text them or leave a short message on their social media page to let them know.

- **Send** cards to people you know who are going through a rough patch in life. A card can make more of a difference than you know.

- **Call** your family regularly and ask them if there is anything that you could do for them, or find out what's going on in their lives that could use some prayers.

"Service to others is the rent you pay for your room here on earth."

Muhammad Ali

STEP 20: Think It Through

Too many people don't think through a plan before they embark on it. Lucy and Ethel (from the *I Love Lucy* show) come to mind when I think of people who never thought through their crazy plans. Lucy always had a plan to do something but never took the time to think it through to the end, and her plans always turned out rather hilarious but kind of sad.

Thinking through a problem means looking at the solutions before allowing the problem to become out of control to the point where it can't be fixed. Artists, writers, engineers, doctors, lawyers, educators, speakers, pastors, marketers, and others do this on a daily basis. They think about problems, sometimes from many angles, before coming up with a solution.

If you look at your life situations, do you ever realize that you're constantly on the "crazy-go-round" of life? Then you're not thinking it through. A crazy-go-round is a life issue that simply won't go away and drives you nuts because no matter what you do or don't do, it never changes.

These crazy-go-rounds may never go away, but as you think these through, they will affect you less and less because you will begin to choose not to focus on them. You'll understand that you can't change the crazy-go-rounds or the other people on them, but you can change yourself and how you think about them.

Thinking through a problem, thinking through a crazy-go-round, thinking through your feelings, thinking through your actions, thinking through your thoughts, and thinking through your choices are the safest ways to live a life filled with wellness.

"Begin with the end in mind."

Stephen Covey

STEP 21: Understanding Your Vision

Sometimes unhealthy issues continue to surface in your life because you don't understand why. "WHY?" This question is asked many times, especially in difficult times.

"Why did this bad thing happen to me?"

"Why did I get this disease?"

"Why did my spouse leave me?"

Then the other half of that question rears its ugly head. "WHY NOT?" The answers to these questions help you to understand the vision you have for your entire life.

While many times you are told not to even think about the question of "Why?" something has happened or is happening in your life. Because people think that you will have to endure even more bad things, just by asking that question. What about the good times? I bet you never think of that question when your life is good, and you're enjoying the moment.

Understanding the vision in your life means that you need to understand the why's and the why not's of the things that happen to you; this means that you need to ask yourself some difficult questions. It's no secret that in order to lose weight and get healthy, you need to ask yourself questions about your motives. Why do you do the deeds that are detrimental to both your figure and your health?

For me, it looks like this: What in my past has me connected to eating chocolate first thing in the morning? This goes all the way back to my grandfather. He cared for my sister and I while my mom worked sometimes. One of his favorite things to give us for breakfast was a cup of coffee with a hunk of chocolate. I long for those simpler times when I was cared for by my Polish grandfather. I feel the need to continue in his legacy even though I know it's not healthy. But in my case, I've changed the way I have my chocolate in the morning and have a chocolate protein shake instead.

I have a vision of looking and feeling a certain way, so I needed to understand why I am constantly craving something that has tied me to my past. Every day you probably do something that you don't know why you're tied to doing it.

Now let's dig a little deeper. I wasn't always a fan of setting goals for myself. I actually had an obsession about not setting goals. When I was much younger, I would set goals only to have them sit on the paper and not get accomplished. After the date I set for my goals came and went, I would focus on the unaccomplished goals instead of the little successes I had. WHY? Because I would let the negative words of my mother overrun my mind instead of focusing on the positive words of my father. Since then, I've accomplished many things in my life by having goals—but those negative words are sometimes so difficult to silence.

You must have a vision of where you want to go in life and what you want to do. But more importantly, you need to understand that vision.

How to understand your vision:

- Write down your goals.

- Read your goals every morning.

- Give your goals an image. What do they look like?

- Surround yourself with photos and quotations that picture your goal.

- Make a vision map for your life.

"The most pathetic person in the world is someone who has sight, but has no vision."

Helen Keller

STEP 22: Visualize Your Dreams

There are some important steps to visualizing what you need to see in order to grow forward and be prosperous in the world. You're not taught these skills in school; they are lessons learned throughout your life.

In fact, you've been taught just the opposite. "Get your head out of the clouds!" "Stop daydreaming!" "You can't believe a hunch!" But sometimes you're told that certain aspects of the visualizing tools are useful, like "a mother's intuition" or "that gut feeling."

Wouldn't it be wonderful if you could use these valid tools to transform all the facets of your life? How would your health be different if you used these tools? You can, and many people already do. You too can learn how to use these tools to help you visualize your dreams.

In the movie *Bedtime Stories*, Adam Sandler's character is an uncle whose niece and nephew had dreams that would come true. So he would implant suggestions to them while he made up bedtime stories. This is what you do when you visualize.

If you're having difficulty visualizing your dreams, then change your paradigms.

Six areas to change:

- **Perception:** How you perceive the world around you has a big impact on how you perceive and visualize your dream. If your perception is based on the premise that everyone is out to get you, then visualizing your dream will not be possible because you will constantly be thinking that someone might take your dream away from you, or someone might be better at what you want to accomplish.

There will always be someone who's better than you. Your competition should be with yourself. Trying to be a better *you* instead of competing with others is a healthier perception than trying to compare yourself with other people.

- **Will:** Do you have the creative ability to carry a mental image of your dream with you at all times? If you can use your imagination to create solutions to problems not yet seen, you can use it to visualize how your dreams came become a reality.

  Get your head back in those clouds and find your imagination again. Use it to bring your dreams to life, to give them form and shape. Only you can bring it to life; you can't rely on your spouse, your parents, or your friends. It's your dream, not theirs.

- **Memory:** Remembering the details of your dream will make going through challenging and mundane tasks easier. Making a dream into a reality is not all roses and glory. It requires that you do tasks you don't like to do and tasks that are just plain menial. But these tasks need to get done so your dream can become a reality. Your memory of what you hold in your mind's eye helps you move forward by motivating you to make changes in your paradigms or your belief systems so they're congruent with the visualization of your dream.

  Changing a belief is as simple as changing the references to it. In order to change the references of a belief system you have to change your thought pattern. Therefore, if you are constantly thinking about the boring tasks and losing sight of your dream, you're not changing your thought patterns or your paradigms. If you adopt a different thought pattern, such as "these mundane tasks will make my dream easier to achieve," your paradigm changes and your dream will become a reality.

- **Intuition:** Your intuition gives you balance. It's what you think about, even when you think you're doing something where you're focusing solely on that one thing. Have you ever been doing something that needed your undivided attention, but in the back of your mind you were thinking something totally incongruent with what you were doing? Have you ever just known that something didn't feel right about a certain situation or place? This is your intuition at work.

  How do you use your intuition to help you visualize your dream? START listening to it. STOP listening to your inner critic that keeps playing in your head, whether the words come from a negative spouse, parent, friend, or even yourself. Stop the words. Stop ridiculing yourself. Write out your thoughts about your dream, the people in your dream, and every other aspect of your dream.

- **Reason:** Can you think logically through a set of steps in order to work out a problem? While visualizing your dream may include many personal emotions that tie you to the dream, you need to get away from the emotions and learn to reason through some points to make your dreams a reality. You have to use sound reasoning skills and prudent judgments when necessary in order to plow through roadblocks that may come up in the pursuit of your dreams.

Notice how all of these tools are all interconnected with each other and with your dreams. Awareness is the first step in using them to visualize what you want in life.

Using these tools will change your paradigms and help in the process of visualizing your dreams, which will propel you forward in your wellness as well as in your life.

"All men dream, but not equally. Those who dream by night in the dusty recesses of their minds, wake in the day to find that it was vanity; but the dreamers of the day are dangerous men, for they may act on their dreams with open eyes, to make them possible."

T. E. Lawrence

STEP 23: Words Shape Your Mind

What we think about, we bring about. Words can either tear you down or build you up, whether you're speaking them out loud or to yourself. Whatever happened to "If you can't say anything nice, don't say anything at all"?

Just like a good diet shapes your health, words shape your mind. If you use the right words, your mind and your world will change accordingly. Many times throughout my day I find myself either repeating quotes or singing words of inspirational music. I quote people who have left a positive stamp on my heart. For me, most of those words come from my father.

"Watch out world, she can do anything she puts her mind to!"

"You have a wonderful heart; you need to let the world see that!"

"Stand in the gap, Laura, it's where people need you the most but are too afraid to ask!"

There are other great motivators who have left their words behind so that you and I can use them to shape our minds.

"You are free to choose, but the choices you make today will determine what you will have, be and do in the tomorrow of your life." ~ Zig Ziglar

"Is prayer your steering wheel or your spare tire?" ~ Corrie Ten Boom

"Any fool can criticize, condemn, and complain—and most fools do. But it takes character and self control to be understanding and forgiving." ~ Dale Carnegie

"I am who I am today because of the choices I made yesterday." ~ Eleanor Roosevelt

"Nothing is impossible with God." ~ Luke 1:37 (New Living Translation)

"A leader's attitude is caught by his or her followers more quickly than his or her actions." ~ John C Maxwell

"I may not be where I need to be, but I thank God I am not where I used to be." ~ Joyce Meyer

"Keep away from people who try to belittle your ambitions. Small people always do that, but the really great make you feel that you, too, can become great." ~ Mark Twain

"Fear does not have any special power unless you empower it by submitting to it." ~ Les Brown

"Change your thoughts and you change your world." ~ Norman Vincent Peale

"You are the building, your words are the bricks, and your thoughts are the mortar. Are you building yourself up or tearing yourself down?"

Laura Jacoby

STEP 24: Waking Up to Exercise

Let's face it, if you don't find exercising fun, many of you won't do it. When does everything in life need to be fun in order to be done? Anyone who's ever changed a diaper knows it's not fun, but it is a necessary part of raising a family. Many other things in life aren't fun, but yet you do them. For some of you, exercise could be in that category.

For people who already love to exercise, this step may be a little boring, but for all of you who dread waking up to exercise and will look for every excuse in the book to not exercise, this post will hit a nerve.

Remember the old saying "use it or lose it"? Well, I have many examples of people in my own life that got no physical activity and their lives were shortened or seriously changed because of this. One such example was my own father. While my father was an inspiring man, his only exercise came when he would walk the trash cans to the end of our driveway. Don't get me wrong—we had all sorts of exercise equipment from stationary bicycles to contraptions that hung on door knobs with leather grips that made you look like you were walking while lying on your back. We also had this one piece of equipment that had four foam pads on a track, two for your hands and two for your knees. It made you feel like you were crawling. Their items were used for about a month, and then they would sit in our basement collecting dust. My father died at the age of 63 back in 1988.

Then I have my uncle Hank. I always remember him as being thin, but he was just as unhealthy as my father when it came to exercising. His favorite exercise was golfing. He loved the sport so much that he had a golfing green installed in his back yard. When I stayed with my aunt and uncle in the summer, I would go golfing with him and we always rode in the golf cart because as he would say, "It took too long to walk it." He died in 1982 at the age of 62.

I have numerous examples in my life of people who would say "I just hate to exercise." "It makes me too sweaty." "I don't like the way I feel when I exercise." "It takes too much time." These are the same people who today are either dead or living in a handicapped state, all because they made excuses about why they didn't do it instead of waking up to exercise.

Your body was not designed to sit all day. It's ironic when you look at it from a mammalian standpoint. You're told that eating organic free-range chickens and organic grass-fed beef is good for you. So the animals are roaming free, and people are sitting in cages.

Now, no amount of eating organic food is going to save a sick population if you're sitting in your own cages that you call offices, homes, and vehicles. If you don't have a physical job, then you better have a physical life. You need to exercise. It's simple—you need to get rid of all the excuses about why you don't exercise. You need to do it whether it's fun or not. Yes, there are all sorts of books and websites out there that tout the benefits of exercising, and you can read them all, but having the knowledge won't make you do it. You just have to wake up, cut the crap, and exercise.

Look for the examples in your own family of people who have really lived, and of those who lived with their excuses. You'll find your motivation to wake up to exercise.

"People spend too much time finding other people to blame, too much energy finding excuses for not being what they are capable of being, and not enough energy putting themselves on the line, growing out of the past, and getting on with their lives."

J. Michael Straczynski

STEP 25: Yearn for Your Own Wellness

Webster's dictionary defines yearning as "a tender or urgent longing." Do you have tenderness and compassion for yourself, where you yearn to make yourself healthy and strong? Do you persistently long after wellness and make your own wellness steps an integral part of your life? It's easier to have compassion for other people, but if you're not yearning for your own wellness, then what are you doing—just playing or dabbling in the wellness pool? You can't consider yourself a swimmer if you're sitting on the side of the pool and only sticking your legs in.

Sometimes I think health and wellness is seen as an afterthought. A busy mom or student might make some of these familiar statements.

"When I have more time, I'll get around to it."

"It's something I'll take more seriously when I'm older."

"I don't need to think about health and wellness. I'm only a teenager (or in my 20s, 30s, or maybe 40s)."

"I'm not sick yet!"

Don't wait for illness and disease to catch you in its grips; you may not have enough time to get out. If you start yearning for your own wellness now, you'll be able to stave off illness, slow down the aging process, lose weight, and be in the best health of your life. Waiting only makes it more difficult.

Be proactively compassionate about your own wellness. Read books, take classes, join groups, communicative effectively, reconnect with loved ones, forgive yourself; do whatever is necessary to show compassion to yourself. If you're willing to treat yourself with compassion, other people will do the same.

"The concept of total wellness recognizes that our every thought, word, and behavior affects our greater health and well-being. And we, in turn are affected not only emotionally but also physically and spiritually."

Greg Anderson

STEP 26: Zip It & Zap It

You're thinking, "What does zip it and zap it have to do with wellness?" So much that you don't even imagine how much, sometimes. These two action steps go together like peanut butter and jelly. If you zip it and zap it, you'll have more days on this earth filled with wellness.

Zip It is a direct relationship to your mouth—not just to foods that make you unhealthy and overweight, but to words that tear down. If your conversation and the words you use are not adding to the encouragement of others, then don't say them. Words are so important. The words you choose can either build a bridge of wellness or leave a legacy of deceit.

When was the last time you were in a conversation with someone and you heard more curse words than anything else? The person using the curse words is filled with strife, contention, and animosity—with others, but more importantly with himself or herself. Learn to control your words for your health's sake. People who don't curse can edify conversations, encourage one another, be calmer, be more at peace, and be healthier than their curse-word-slinging counterparts.

Zap It is entirely connected to the negative energy that's produced by negative people, negative situations, negative words, and negative thoughts. If you are yearning for better wellness, then you'll want to zap all the areas that are negative in your own lives.

Just like the microwave zaps all the nutrients out of your food, you need to zap all the negative influences that cause you strife. Granted, you probably can't do anything about the traffic you drive in every day, but you can alter your response to it.

Ways to Zap It (remove the negative energy)

- **Get away** from negative people. If you're married to someone who is constantly negative, then find your happy place in your mind and go there when your spouse is in a negative mood. Talk to your spouse and ask why he or she is negative all the time. Seek counseling, if necessary. Find something that the two of you like to do and make a commitment to do it at least once a month. If the negative person is your boss, find your happy place, and if the situation is bleak, find another job (on your own time).

- **Stop** using negative words yourself. Zip your mouth if you can't say anything nice to someone. Hold yourself to a higher standard. Don't let the negative words of others spur you into a negative world. If you praise your children for what they are doing right instead of constantly criticizing them for all the mistakes they make, they will be happier and will want to do better instead of not wanting to try at all.

- **Create** a list of positive words to say every day. It sounds childish, but you are learning a new habit, you may need a little bit of prompting throughout the day. (See Appendix A for my positive word list.)

- **Stop** watching television shows and movies that encourage negativity. When you're in a negative place watching movies about arguments, killings, and evil, it will only fuel the fire within you.

- **Stop** eating junk food. Junk food is filled with negative energy and needs to zap too many nutrients from your body just to digest it. Instead, choose live food—nothing packaged with a label or purchased from a fast food restaurant. Eat an orange, a banana, an organic piece of chicken, or a salad. Choose as many organic foods as you can that give you positive energy. The longer a person runs on negative energy, the higher their risk of contracting deadly diseases.

- **Keep** a notebook with you. When you're going through a negative situation, write down your thoughts about it. Then cross out the negative thoughts and write down something positive about the situation. Write something positive about being stuck in traffic. Write something positive about crazy-go-round family issues. Write something positive about all the negative situations in your life, and you'll begin to see those same situations as positive opportunities for growth.

"Bondage is – subjection to external influences and internal negative thoughts and attitudes."

W. Clement Stone

Appendix A: Laura's Positive Word List

Good	Rejoice
Great	Ecstatic
Awesome	Approve
Magnificent	Believe
Inspiring	Beautiful
Encouraging	Fabulous
Absolutely	Fantabulous
Delight	Fantastic
Generous	Ideal
Laughter	Happy
Quality	Honorable
Terrific	Marvelous

Notes

1. O.G. Mouritsen, *Life – As a Matter of Fat: The Emerging Science of Lipidomics* (Berlin: Springer-Verlag, 2006), 175.

2. G.L. Samuelson, G. L., *The Science of Healing Revealed: New Insights into Redox Signaling* (Sandy, Utah: Gary Samuelson, 2009), 56.

3. L. Skidmore-Roth, *Mosby's Handbook of Herbs & Natural Supplements, 4th ed.* (St. Louis, MO: Mosby Elsevier, 2010), 241–243.

4. L. Skidmore-Roth, *Mosby's Handbook of Herbs & Natural Supplements, 4th ed.* (St. Louis, MO: Mosby Elsevier, 2010), 260–263.

5. L. Skidmore-Roth, *Mosby's Handbook of Herbs & Natural Supplements, 4th ed.* (St. Louis, MO: Mosby Elsevier, 2010), 263–265.

6. L. Skidmore-Roth, *Mosby's Handbook of Herbs & Natural Supplements, 4th ed.* (St. Louis, MO: Mosby Elsevier, 2010), 281–285.

7. J. A. Duke, *The Green Pharmacy Guide to Healing Foods* (New York: Rodale, 2008), 339.

8. L. Skidmore-Roth, *Mosby's Handbook of Herbs & Natural Supplements, 4th ed.* (St. Louis, MO: Mosby Elsevier, 2010), 473–475.

9. Allergy Adapt, Inc. (http://www.food-allergy.org/spelt.html, 2011).

10. J.F. Balch & M. Stengler, *Prescription for Natural Cures* (Hoboken, NJ: John Wiley & Sons, 2004), 102.

11. J.F. Balch & M. Stengler, *Prescription for Natural Cures* (Hoboken, NJ: John Wiley & Sons, 2004), 218–223.

12. J.F. Balch & M. Stengler, *Prescription for Natural Cures* (Hoboken, NJ: John Wiley & Sons, 2004), 251–256.

13. J.F. Balch & M. Stengler, *Prescription for Natural Cures* (Hoboken, NJ: John Wiley & Sons, 2004), 220.

14. J. Mercola (http://articles.mercola.com/sites/articles/archive/2010/11/22/how-ultraprocessed-foods-are-killing-us.aspx, 2010).

Recommended Reading

Blaylock, R. *Excitotoxins: The Taste That Kills*. Santa Fe, NM: Health Press, 1996.

Carnegie, D. *How to Stop Worrying & Start Living*. New York: Galahad, 1998.

Covey, S.R. *The 7 Habits of Highly Effective People*. New York: Simon & Schuster, 1989.

Fuhrman, J. *Eat to Live*. New York: Hachette Book Group, 2011.

Gilbere, G. *Chemical Cuisine: Do You REALLY Know What You're Eating?* Sandpoint, ID: IWR, 2011

Leaf, C. *Who Switched Off My Brain? Controlling Toxic Thoughts and Emotions*. USA: Thomas Nelson, 2009.

Maxwell, J.C. *Thinking for a Change: 11 Ways Highly Successful People Approach Life and Work*. New York: Warner Books, 2003.

Meyer, J. *Change Your Words, Change Your Life*. New York: Hachette Book Group, 2012.

Mindell, E & Hopkins, V. *Prescription Alternatives: Hundreds of Safe, Natural, Prescription-Free Remedies to Restore and Maintain Your Health*. New York: McGraw-Hill, 2009.

Pollan, M. *The Omnivore's Dilemma: A Natural History of Four Meals*. New York: Penguin, 2006.

Reynolds, G. *The First 20 Minutes: Surprising Science Reveals How We Can Exercise Better, Train Smarter, and Live Longer*. New York: Penguin, 2013.

Robbins, A. *Awaken The Giant Within*. New York: Free Press, 2003.

Smith, J. *Seeds of Deception: Exposing Industry and Government Lies about the Safety of the Genetically Engineered Foods You're Eating*. Fairfield, IA: Yes Books, 2003.

Tracy, B. *Goals: How to Get Everything You Want—Faster Than You Ever Thought Possible*. San Francisco: Berrett-Koehler, 2010.

Ziglar, Z. *See You At The Top: 25th Anniversary Edition*. Gretna, LA: Pelican, 2000.

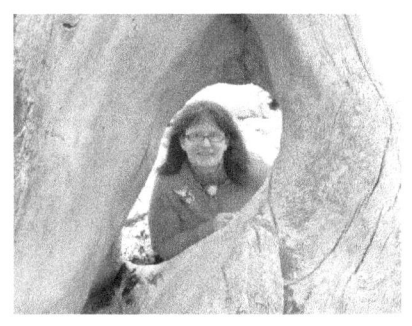

About the Author

Laura Jacoby was born in Chicago, Illinois and grew up in Munster, IN. She is the youngest of four children. Laura's interest in health grew from the examples of her parents and many aunts and uncles who died too young. Laura married her best friend in 1985 and had four wonderful sons in three years. As if raising her brood wasn't a full time job, Laura ran several businesses, homeschooled her sons for a bit and eventually took a job working in the school district her sons attended. When all of her sons were grown, Laura entertained the notion of going to college. She began her college career in 2008 and graduated with honors in 2012 with a Bachelor of Science degree in Health & Wellness. Laura enjoys camping, hiking, cooking, foraging, singing in choir, reading, crocheting, writing, and most of all, spending time with her husband and family.

Visit Laura's wellness blog at http://well2day.me/.

Photography Credits (cover and author): Harbor Joe Photos